FLAXSEEDS AN ANTIDOTE TO GUT PROBLEMS

YOUR SHIELD AGAINST BREAST CANCER

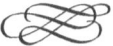

MARTIN EDEN

CONTENTS

INTRODUCTION

Seems like every Christmas we hear about people camping out for several days in advance of a "doorbuster" event on Black Friday.

The stores run such crazy good deals that people brave the cold and live in tents for days. It's not just Christmas. Kids also line up in long queues to get new books in the Harry Potter series. Same thing with whenever Apple releases some new whiz bag gadget – people will camp out to make sure they're first in line to buy it.

You know what? Getting a book or gadget first isn't exactly a life-changing experience, and yet it means enough to the person that they're willing to suffer to get what they want.

So let me ask you...

What would you do to get relief from your gut problems or protect yourself against breast cancer? If you have ever had either of these challenges, you've probably suffered so much that you won't mind using natural treatments (such as Flaxseeds) rather than surgical procedures.

The truth is, there's a lot of contradictory and sometimes,

outright false information floating around about this topic. Hence, we rolled up our sleeves to show you:

- Top 10 reasons why you should eat more flaxseed
- How Flaxseeds work for weight loss
- The relationship between flaxseeds and breast cancer
- 10 healthy ways to consume flaxseeds
- 5 proven home remedies for constipation using Flaxseeds
- Flaxseed's smoothie recipes, breakfast recipes, bread recipes, soup recipes, oatmeal recipes, cookie recipes, and snack recipes

Without further introduction, let's start with the *"Top 10 Reasons Why You Should Eat More Flaxseed."*

TOP 10 REASONS WHY YOU SHOULD EAT MORE FLAXSEED

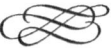

*F*laxseeds have been in existence for ages and are continuously being utilized because they have protective health characteristics.

It is well documented that Charles the great and his subordinates consume Flaxseeds regularly. Hence, gave it the name "the most useful" (in Latin: Linum Usitatissimum)

Advancements in scientific research have highlighted the other benefits of Flaxseeds.

Here are the top 10 of such benefits:

1. Flaxseeds are highly nutritious

Flaxseeds are one of the oldest crops grown since the start of civilization. Both the brown and golden types of flaxseeds have equal amounts of nutrients. One tablespoon (7 grams) is the typical serving size for ground Flaxseeds, and this serving size is a rich source of vitamins, minerals, protein, fiber, and omega-3 fatty acids.

The fiber, lignin, and omega-3 fatty acids are the main reasons why Flaxseeds are highly beneficial to your health.

. . .

2. Flaxseeds are rich in omega-3 fats

Especially if you don't eat fish or you are a vegetarian. Flaxseeds contain large amounts of alpha-linolenic acid (ALA) which is a rich source of omega-3 fatty acid. Since the human body can't produce 'ALA,' you have to obtain it from the food you eat. Research has proven that the ALA in Flaxseeds can cause a reduction in tumor growth, reduction in the inflammation of the arteries and prevention of cholesterol deposition in your heart's blood vessels.

3. Flaxseeds may reduce cancer risk because they are rich in lignins

Though they are plant compounds, lignins can reduce the risk of cancer because they have estrogen and antioxidant properties.

Apart from preventing cancer in premenopausal women, evidence has also shown that most postmenopausal women can be at a lower risk of breast cancer when they consume Flaxseeds.

Men who consume up to 30 grams of flaxseeds per day in a low-fat diet are at a lower risk of prostate cancer. This diet reduces the levels of the marker for prostate cancer. Some lab studies have indicated that Flaxseeds can help prevent colon and skin cancers. It is safe to conclude that Flaxseeds are super foods that can prevent any cancer.

More about this benefit will be discussed in the next chapter.

4. Flaxseeds improve bowel movements since they are a rich source of dietary fiber

Soluble and insoluble dietary fibers are the two types in

Flaxseeds. However, both can be fermented by bacteria to bulk stools and improve bowel movements. Soluble fiber lowers your digestion rate by increasing the consistency in the contents of your intestine. Thus, lowering your cholesterol and regulating your blood sugar levels.

But insoluble fibers increases bulk stools by allowing more water to bind to them and softening your stools. Hence, those with diverticular disease or irritable bowel syndrome can avoid constipation.

5. Flaxseeds help to lower cholesterol levels

The fiber in Flaxseeds can bind to bile salts which makes it easily excreted out of your body. Then, cholesterol is drawn from your blood into your liver to replenish the lost bile salts. Thus, your cholesterol blood levels are reduced. If you desire a reduction in your cholesterol levels, this is one of your best options.

6. Flaxseeds can reduce blood pressure

Apart from decreasing the blood pressure of those with uncontrollable high blood pressure, Flaxseeds further reduce the blood pressure of those taking blood pressure medication.

7. Flaxseeds supply an abundance quantity of plant-based protein

The flaxseed protein contains copious amounts of amino acids such as glutamic acid, aspartic acid, and arginine. According to research, this flaxseed protein has anti-fungal properties, prevents tumors, lower cholesterol, and improve immune function.

If you desire to reduce your meat intake without worrying

about being hungry, Flaxseeds may be your best option. It provides the same benefits you will get from consuming animal protein.

8. Flaxseeds can reduce blood sugar levels

The insoluble fiber content in Flaxseeds makes it possible for it to reduce blood sugar levels. It is a proven fact that insoluble fiber reduces blood sugar levels because it can lower the release of sugar into your bloodstream.

Bear in mind that if you consume flaxseed oil, you won't enjoy this benefit. There is no fiber in flaxseed oil. If you have diabetes, adding Flaxseeds can be beneficial and nutritious to you.

9. Flaxseeds help you to fend off hunger pangs

The soluble fiber content in Flaxseeds is credited for reducing hunger feelings. By triggering the hormones that control appetite and provide a feeling of satisfaction, it slows down digestion in your stomach.

By reducing hunger feelings but increasing feelings of satiation, the dietary content in Flaxseeds may assist in weight control.

10. You can consume Flaxseeds in a lot of ways

The details will be discussed in the chapter after the next chapter. To preserve its freshness, you should consume Flaxseeds ground with a coffee grinder rather than the whole.

FLAXSEED OIL: WHAT YOU SHOULD KNOW

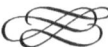

*T*he nutritional properties and the health benefits of flaxseed oil have contributed to its increased popularity in recent times. The cold pressing process is the typical way to extract flax seed oil. It is best for you to keep flaxseed oil in the dark glass bottles and store it in a dark and cool place to preserve its nutritional benefits. Flaxseed oil is not usually used for high-temperature cooking because some of its nutrients are sensitive to heat.

However, at 177 degrees C./350 degrees F., there is virtually no difference in the quality of flaxseed oil.

The alpha-linolenic acid (ALA) concentrations are one major difference between flaxseed oil and Flaxseeds. There are 7 grams of in 7 grams of ALA in one tablespoon of flaxseed oil, while one tablespoon of ground Flaxseeds contains 1.6 grams of 'ALA.'

Ground Flaxseeds are your best choice to enjoy the full health benefits of Flaxseeds. To prevent abuse, experts recommend that you should not consume more than five tablespoons of Flaxseeds daily.

Flaxseed oil can interact with antiplatelet medications since it can decrease platelet aggregation. Also, flaxseed oil can cause very low blood pressure since it can lower blood sugar. Hence, don't take flaxseed oil with blood pressure medication unless you have sought permission from your doctor. This precaution is also applicable to any new supplement.

To avoid mild hormonal effects, experts recommend that you should avoid taking flaxseed oil and flaxseed when you are pregnant.

DIFFERENCE BETWEEN FLAXSEED AND FLAXSEED OIL: WHICH OF THEM IS BETTER?

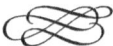

*T*he nutritional content in ground flaxseed and flaxseed oil is different. Hence, they offer various health benefits.

CALORIES AND FIBER

Ground flaxseed contains more fiber but fewer calories than flaxseed oil. Two tablespoons of flaxseed oil contain 240 calories while two tablespoons of ground flaxseed contain 75 calories.

There is no fiber in flaxseed oil, but one serving of ground flaxseed contains 3.8 grams of dietary fiber. Dietary fiber is known to cause satiation and boost cardiovascular health.

Also, if you're a man, taking one serving of ground flaxseed provides you with 10 percent of your daily fiber intake. And if you're a woman, taking one serving of ground flaxseed provides you with 15 percent of your daily fiber intake.

Omega-3 fatty acids

There are more omega-3 fatty acids in a serving of flaxseed oil than a serving of ground flaxseeds. A diet rich in omega-3 fatty acids boosts brain function, maintains your heart's health and prevent omega-3 fatty acid deficiency (which is known to cause depression and dry skin).

A 2-tablespoon of ground flaxseed contains 3.2 grams of 'ala,' while the same quantity of serving for flaxseed oil contains 14.6 grams of ALA. Men need just 1.5 grams of ALA per day, while women need 1.1 grams. This dietary content is provided in one serving of flaxseed oil.

MINERAL COMPOSITION

There is no significant quantity of minerals in flaxseed oil, but each serving of ground flaxseed contains 171 micrograms of copper and 55 milligrams of magnesium. Copper controls the production of energy, while magnesium boosts the proper functioning of your muscles.

Lignin boost

Apart from regulating estrogen in your body, ground flaxseed can also prevent genetic mutations and cellular damage. Ground flaxseed improves your lignin consumption, but flaxseed oil separates the lignins in flaxseed from the fats.

To enjoy the full benefits of lignins and other nutrients, it is best you consume flaxseed oil which also includes ground flaxseed.

THE RELATIONSHIP BETWEEN FLAXSEEDS AND BREAST CANCER

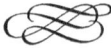

HOW FLAXSEEDS PREVENT BREAST CANCER

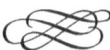

*Y*ou can protect yourself from breast cancer having breast cancer by consuming high amounts of lignin. Due to its lignin content, flaxseed has become one major ingredient you should include in your diet to prevent breast cancer, prevent the recurrence of breast cancer or improve your chances of surviving breast cancer.

However, high concentrations of lignin are mostly found in berries, fruits, vegetables, whole grains, and seeds. Hence, if you consume lots of veggies, you are consuming at least eight times more lignin content than others.

Researchers from the University of Kansas subjected women who are highly susceptible to breast cancer "one teaspoon of ground flaxseeds per day for one year." They observed that there was a reduction in the precancerous changes in their breasts.

Another study published in cancer causes and control showed that an average of 25 percent reduction in breast cancer risk could be attributed to the daily consumption of flaxseed. Hence, by consuming small amounts of flaxseed daily, you will have sufficient quantities of lignin in your body that will reduce your risk of having breast cancer.

HOW FLAXSEEDS HELP YOU TO
SURVIVE BREAST CANCER

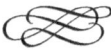

*N*ew research evidence suggests that women with breast cancer who consume high amounts of lignin live longer than those who don't. The lignins prevent cancer cell migration and inhibit the growth of breast cancer cells.

Some University of Toronto researchers discovered that within four weeks, flax reduced the growth of tumor in the human breast.

HOW FLAXSEEDS CONTRIBUTE TO BREAST CANCER PROTECTION

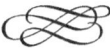

The four ways flaxseeds contribute to breast cancer protection are:

• They supply your body with large amounts of omega-3 fatty acids which boosts your immunes against the growth of breast cancer cells

• They prevent constipation (a cause of breast cancer) because they can move stool out of your body at the right time due to their mucilaginous (slippery) properties.

• They bind and push out hormones and carcinogens which aids breast cancer

• They prevent inflammation. Flaxseeds aids the generation of interleukin-1 receptor antagonist molecule which prevents the production of interleukin-1 - a molecule responsible for the feeding, growth, and invasion of tumors.

Research shows that consuming flax for one month can increase the levels of interleukin-1 receptor antagonist in your body by at least 50 percent. Though the removal of breasts or ovaries and the consumption of tamoxifen drug can prevent generation of estrogen receptor (which is a major cause of breast cancer) are effective, they are costly and have serious side effects such as blood clots and uterine cancer.

However, Flaxseeds' lignins do not only improve breast cancer survival but also decrease your susceptibility to breast cancer.

HOW LIGNINS PREVENT CANCEROUS GROWTH

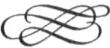

*E*nterolignins can bind to estrogen receptors because they have a similar structure to estrogen. However, there is a gradual reduction of enterolignins in your gut due to the presence of antibiotics which are capable of destroying beneficial bacteria in your gut.

Two common sources of antibiotics are commercial meats, overuse and inappropriate consumption of antibiotic drugs.

THE THREE BEST SOURCES OF
PLANT LIGNINS

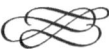

Flaxseeds, chia seeds, and sesame seeds are the three best sources of plant lignins. However, flaxseeds contain the highest amount of lignin content. Its content is three times more than that of chia seeds and eight times more than that of sesame seeds. Conversely, there are no lignins in flaxseed oil since it binds to the fiber.

Below is the lignin content of plant foods that contain lignin:

- Flaxseeds (85.5 mg/ounce)
- Chia seeds (32 mg/ounce)
- Sesame seeds (11.2 mg/ounce)
- Kale (curly; 1.6 mg/cup)
- Broccoli (1.2 mg/cup)

Enterolignins lower serum estrogen levels since they inhibit the production of aromatase and estradiol. Also, plant lignins bind globulin (thus, blunts the effects of estrogen) but increase the concentration of sex hormone. You can significantly reduce your susceptibility to breast cancer by combining your daily intake of ground Flaxseeds with your greens, beans, mushrooms, and onions.

HOW FLAXSEEDS WORK FOR WEIGHT LOSS

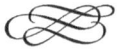

*B*ased on its molecular composition and nutritional properties such as being rich in lignin, fiber, and omega-3 acids, Flaxseeds can aid weight loss.

However, note that:

• Flaxseeds require a healthy diet and an exercise plan to work effectively

• Your weight loss results may vary since your body's reaction to flaxseed supplements won't be the same with the others.

There are two common ways to use Flaxseeds for weight loss:

1. A drink

Flaxseeds in weight loss drinks improve digestion, makes you feel full for long periods, and boosts your metabolism. You'll need ground Flaxseeds to make your drink. You can either purchase one or buy whole flaxseeds, then, grind them.

Here's how to prepare this drink:

Ingredients

tsp freshly ground flax seed

lemon wedge

4 oz. hot water

Instructions

Stir the ground flax seed in hot water. Squeeze the lemon wedge (this adds vitamin c and some flavor to your drink). For optimum results, it is best you take this drink once daily.

2. As an oral supplement

Oral flaxseed supplements containing pressed flaxseed oil are easier to consume than those containing raw Flaxseeds. Also, for the best results, you're required to take these supplements once daily.

PRECAUTIONS TO TAKE BEFORE YOU USE FLAXSEEDS TO LOSE WEIGHT

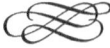

• *A*void unripe or raw Flaxseeds. They contain toxic substances and can cause indigestion.

• Although there is no evidence to support taking Flaxseeds as a nursing mother, you should avoid taking Flaxseeds when you're pregnant to avoid hormonal side effects.

• Regardless of the form in which you are consuming Flaxseeds, always drink lots of water when taking it. Otherwise, your body won't digest the excess fiber properly. Thus, leading to constipation and stomach cramps

OTHER HEALTH BENEFITS OF FLAXSEEDS

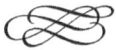

*A*part from aiding weight loss and reducing the risk of some cancers, Flaxseeds are also useful for:
- Supporting a healthy kidney
- Improving digestion
- Lowering cholesterol

PURCHASING FLAXSEEDS

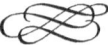

ost of the health food stores, grocery stores in your neighborhood and dietary supplement sellers will sell ground Flaxseeds, pure flaxseed oil, and flaxseed oil capsules. If or when they don't have, you can purchase from Amazon or any other online retailer.

13 HEALTHY WAYS TO CONSUME FLAXSEEDS

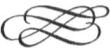

*R*eduction of cholesterol and prevention of cancer are two of the most common benefits of flaxseeds. However, you can only obtain the maximum benefits from flaxseeds when you ground it and store in a refrigerator in this ground form.

Here are ten proven ways to boost recipes with this superfood:

1. Top your oatmeal or yogurt

This is the real secret to consuming flaxseeds daily. It is also a healthy way to begin your day. You can also mix any of your daily recipes with one tablespoon of ground flaxseeds.

2. Improve the nutrients of your soups

Create a velvety and nutty finish in your soups by replacing most of the butter or cream in your creamy soup with two tablespoons of ground flaxseeds. You can also add a small number of whole flaxseeds to create a pop color and crunch finish in your soups. You can replace the cream of any creamy, dreamy soup recipes with the ground flaxseed.

3. Create a sufficient healthy fat

Flaxseeds and sunflower seeds contain sufficient healthy fats to provide your body with a nutritious creamy and buttery spread. To avoid the unappealing taste of flaxseed butter, start by adding ground flaxseeds to your favorite nut spread such as peanut butter.

4. Provide additional nutrition to your salad dressings

Iron, copper, calcium, selenium, zinc, manganese, magnesium, and phosphorus are some of the copious amounts of minerals in flaxseeds. Hence, boost the nutrition in your salad dressings by swirling ground flaxseeds over it.

5. An addition to your vegetarian burger recipe

Create a meaty flavor in your vegetarian burger recipe by adding flaxseeds to it. Thus, you can save some cash or join the Meatless Monday group. Since flaxseeds can hold ingredients together and are gluten-free, you can replace the breadcrumbs in recipes with a quarter cup of ground flaxseeds.

6. Create more nutritious bread, cakes, cookies, and muffins

If you love crispy, crunchy breaded chicken nuggets, you can create better bread by replacing two tablespoons of flour in a cup of the flour with two tablespoons of ground flaxseeds.

You can replace two tablespoons of the flour in zucchini fries and coconut shrimp with two tablespoons of ground flaxseeds. Also, you can add ground Flaxseeds to the mixture for your cakes, cookies, bread, and muffins.

· · ·

7. As a replacement for eggs

Whether or not you're allergic to eggs or vegan, you can perform this swap. It is a proven fact that the mixture of flaxseeds and water creates a liquid mixture similar to eggs. Hence, if you've exhausted your eggs or you don't want to use eggs, you can mix ground flaxseeds with water in the ratio 1-part ground flaxseeds to 3 parts water. Set the mixture aside till you gather the remaining ingredients.

8. Swap the oils

Want to reduce your blood cholesterol? Include at least three tablespoons of flaxseeds in your daily diet. Hence, use three tablespoons of ground flaxseeds in place of one tablespoon oil. Rather than use cup oil in a recipe, use cup oil and cup ground flaxseeds.

9. Increase the dietary fiber content of your favorite granola

Though it is recommended that you consume up 35 grams of dietary fiber per day, if you are like most Americans, you are not fulfilling this recommendation. To fulfill this recommendation, add at between 2 and four tablespoons of ground flaxseeds in your granola. It is proven that there are 4 grams of dietary fiber in two tablespoons of flaxseeds.

10. Blend some into your favorite smoothie recipes

Flaxseeds contain omega-3 fatty acids which are beneficial for the health of your heart. Include at least two tablespoons in some of your smoothies to increase the healthy fat you consume. You can either pulse two tablespoons of flaxseeds and refrigerate or buy ground flaxseeds from the store in your neighborhood.

The next chapter contains some healthy smoothie recipes for your consumption.

11. Add to your morning cereal
Sprinkle ground flaxseeds over cold cereal or stir them in your oatmeal or any other hot cereal.

12. Boost the nutrient in your salad
Top your salad with whole or ground flax oil to enjoy an omega-3 and fiber-rich vinaigrette for your salad.

13. Dressing for your proteins
Add ground flaxseeds to the dressing of your tuna, chicken or egg salad.

5 PROVEN HOME REMEDIES FOR CONSTIPATION USING FLAXSEEDS

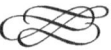

*R*esearch has proven that flaxseed is effective for treating constipation because it can hasten movements within your intestine. Thus, increasing the frequency of your bowel movements.

For the best results, drink plenty of water when consuming any of these home remedies.

REMEDY 1:

Pulse equal parts of the sesame seeds, sunflower seeds, almonds, and Flaxseeds. Add one tablespoon of this mixture to your morning cereal, juice, smoothie or evening salad

This mixture provides your body with the right amounts of minerals and fiber. Flaxseeds are effective for moderate symptoms of constipation. Don't consume more than three cups of flaxseeds per day. Otherwise, it will toxify your colon since it contains small amounts of prussic acid which can become excessive when you consume excess amounts of flaxseed.

.   .   .

REMEDY 2:

Stir one tablespoon of ground flaxseed in 10 ounces of water; set aside for one hour. Drink this mixture before going to bed. Then, drink an equal amount of water.

REMEDY 3:

Add one tablespoon of ground flaxseed to two cups of boiling distilled water. Continue boiling till mixture is jelly-like. Switch off the heat, wait for it to cool. Then, drizzle a teaspoon of apple cider vinegar. Drink a cup of this mixture every morning till you're comfortable with your bowel movement.

Remedy 4:

Stir in one tablespoon each of oat bran and flax seed in one glass of distilled water. Set aside all night; take two tablespoons of this mixture before you eat anything in the morning. Also, wait half an hour before eating anything.

Repeat each morning till your bowels start moving.

REMEDY 5:

Combine one tablespoon each of flaxseed oil, yogurt and a pinch of honey. Add water to desired thickness. Take a glass of this mixture 30 minutes before going to bed. Do not refrigerate or heat flaxseed oil; it can release cancer-causing compounds in your body

SMOOTHIE RECIPES, BREAKFASTS, SNACKS, SOUPS, COOKIES

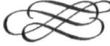

YOGURT FLAXSEED SMOOTHIE

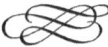

*P*rep time: 7 mins., total time: 7 min.
Serves: 2

Ingredients:

- orange, peeled
- 2 oz. Plain Greek yogurt
- tsp vanilla extract
- 2 tsp flaxseed meal
- 1 cup ice

Instructions:

Pulse all ingredients till smooth

Nutritional information:

Calories 57, fat 1.2g, cholesterol 3mg, sodium 17mg, carbs. 7.3g, dietary fiber 1.7g, sugars 5.3g, protein 3.7g

BANANA APPLE SMOOTHIE

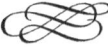

*P*rep time: 5 mins., total time: 5 min.
Serves: 3

Ingredients:
- cup water
- cup oat milk
- cup oats
- cup nonfat vanilla yogurt
- 1 tsp chia seeds
- 2 tsp ground Flaxseeds
- apple, cored and sliced
- banana, frozen
- tsp cinnamon
- tsp nutmeg
- 7 ice cubes

INSTRUCTIONS:

Blend all ingredients with a high-speed blender for 1 minute.

Nutritional information:

Calories 170, fat 4.7g, cholesterol 1mg, sodium 32mg, carbs. 28.5g, dietary fiber 6.9g, sugars 10.1g, protein 5.3g

RASPBERRY FLAXSEED SMOOTHIE

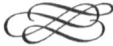

*P*rep time: 5 mins., total time: 5 min.
Serves: 2

Ingredients:
- cup fresh raspberries
- 2 tsp ground flaxseed
- ripe mango, peeled and cubed
- cup low-fat Greek yogurt

Instructions:
1. Blend all ingredients to desired smoothness
2. Serve in glasses and top with fresh raspberries

Nutritional information:
Calories 109, fat 1.6g, cholesterol 2mg, sodium 18mg, carbs. 22.6g, dietary fiber 4g, sugars 18.6g, protein 2.7g

STRAWBERRY FLAX SMOOTHIE

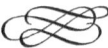

*P*rep time: 5 mins., total time: 5 min.
Serves: 4

Ingredients:

cup strawberry yogurt

cup plain yogurt

6 strawberries, cubed

2 tbsp. Flaxseed, ground

Instructions:

Blend all ingredients to desired smoothness

NUTRITIONAL INFORMATION:

Calories 80, fat 2.7g, cholesterol 3mg, sodium 37mg, carbs. 8.4g, dietary fiber 2.6g, sugars 4.9g, protein 4g

CINNAMON FLAX SMOOTHIE

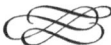

*P*rep time: 5 mins., total time: 5 min.
Serves: 3

Ingredients:
- 1 tbsp. Cinnamon
- cup non-fat yogurt
- 1 tsp. Coffee powder
- banana
- 2 tsp flaxseed, ground

Instructions:
Blend all ingredients using a high-speed blender till smooth
Nutritional information:
Calories 94, fat 0.6g, cholesterol 2mg, sodium 81mg, carbs. 20.2g, dietary fiber 2.1g, sugars 10g, protein 2.4g

PINEAPPLE ORANGE FLAX SMOOTHIE

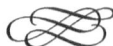

*P*rep time: 10 mins., total time: 10 min.
Serves: 4

Ingredients:

- 2 tbsp. Flaxseed, ground
- 1 cup frozen pineapple
- 2 cups orange juice
- 1 large bunch spinach
- 1 frozen ripe banana, peeled
- 1 cup strawberry

GARNISHING:

- 1 serving shredded dried mulberries

Instructions:

Blend all ingredients using a high-speed blender till smooth

Note: blend the fresh ingredients before adding the frozen ingredients

Nutritional information:

Calories 178, fat 2.7g, cholesterol 0mg, sodium 71mg, carbs. 35.1g, dietary fiber 4.6g, sugars 25.7g, protein 4.9g

BANANA FLAX SMOOTHIE

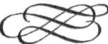

*P*rep time: 10 mins., total time: 10 min.
Serves: 2

Ingredients:
- cup fresh orange juice
- banana, peeled and cubed
- 2 ice cubes
- cup vanilla yogurt
- tsp nutritional yeast
- tbsp. flaxseed oil
- tbsp. wheat germ

INSTRUCTIONS:

1. Blend all ingredients using a high-speed blender till smooth

2. Refrigerate and serve cold in tall glasses

Nutritional information:

Calories 113, fat 4.2g, cholesterol 2mg, sodium 24mg, carbs. 15.9g, dietary fiber 1.1g, sugars 11g, protein 2.8g

BLUEBERRY CINNAMON FLAX PANCAKES

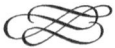

*P*rep time: 5 mins., cook time: 20 mins. Total time: 25 min.

Serves: 6

Ingredients:

- cup whole wheat pastry flour
- 1 cup flaxseed, ground
- 1 small egg
- 1 tbsp. Cinnamon
- tsp sea salt
- 2 tsp baking powder
- 2 tsp vanilla extract
- cup coconut milk
- 1 cup blueberries
- tbsp. Olive oil

INSTRUCTIONS:

1. Stir all dry ingredients in a large bowl
2. Stir all wet ingredients in a separate bowl
3. Stir in cup blueberries gradually

4. Stir the wet and dry ingredients together (presence of small lumps is allowed)

5. Cook each side over medium heat till crispy

6. Top with the remaining blueberries; serve warm

NUTRITIONAL INFORMATION:

Calories 291, fat 19.8g, cholesterol 23mg, sodium 101mg, carbs. 20.9g, dietary fiber 8.4g, sugars 4.6g, protein 6.6g

FLAXSEED WRAPS

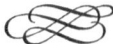

*P*rep time: 10 mins., cook time: 5 mins., total time: 15 min.

Serves: 4

Ingredients:
- 6 tbsp. Flaxseed, ground
- tsp baking powder
- 2 tbsp. Coconut oil
- 2 large eggs
- cup water

INSTRUCTIONS:

1. Blend all ingredients to smooth consistency
2. Pour mixture in a greased microwave-safe bowl
3. Microwave till cooked (about 5 minutes)
4. Remove from microwave and allow to cool (an additional 5 minutes)
5. Take off the wrap from the bowl by gently lifting an edge of the wrap using a spatula

6. Flip over the wrap; garnish with your favorite toppings

Nutritional information:

Calories 150, fat 12.6g, cholesterol 93mg, sodium 39mg, carbs. 3.5g, dietary fiber 2.9g, sugars 0.3g, protein 5.1g

GRANOLA WITH LEMON CURD

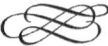

*P*rep time: 10 mins., total time: 10 min.
Serves: 3

Ingredients:
- 5 tbsp. Vanilla yogurt
- 5 tbsp. Lemon curd
- 5 tbsp. Granola
- 6 cup, halves Fresh Fruit
- 3 tbsp. Flaxseed, ground

INSTRUCTIONS:
1. Blend all ingredients to a smooth consistency
2. Split mixture into two glasses
3. Top each glass with Flaxseeds; Eat at once

Nutritional information:

Calories 158, fat 9.6g, cholesterol 2mg, sodium 26mg, carbs. 32.8g, dietary fiber 4.2g, sugars 7g, protein 6.5g

OAT CURRANT FLAX DISH

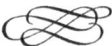

*P*rep time: 10 mins., cook time: 10 min., total time: 20 min.

Serves: 4

Ingredients:
- 5 cups water
- serving quick cooking oats
- cup currants
- tsp ground cinnamon
- cup ground flaxseed
- 1 tbsp. Maple syrup

INSTRUCTIONS:

1. Boil water over high heat in a medium saucepan
2. Stir in the cinnamon, currants, and oats
3. Lower the heat, simmer for 5 minutes; stir once
4. Stir the ground flaxseed, top with the syrup and serve!

. . .

NUTRITIONAL INFORMATION:

Calories 269, fat 9.8g, cholesterol 0mg, sodium 17mg, carbs. 34.2g, dietary fiber 8.9g, sugars 4.4g, protein 8.1g

BANANA GREEK YOGURT

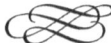

*P*rep time: 10 mins., total time: 10 min.
Serves: 6

Ingredients:

- 3 cups vanilla Greek yogurt
- 3 medium bananas, peeled and sliced
- cup creamy peanut butter
- cup flax seed meal
- 2 tsp nutmeg, ground

INSTRUCTIONS:

1. Split the yogurt into four bowls and add banana slices to each bowl

2. Microwave the peanut butter till it's melted (about 40 seconds); sprinkle one tablespoon of the melted peanut butter on each bowl

3. Add the flax seed and the ground nutmeg

4. Mix thoroughly; serve

Nutritional information:

Calories 345, fat 16.2g, cholesterol 10mg, sodium 135mg, carbs. 35.4g, dietary fiber 5.5g, sugars 20.9g, protein 17.1g

CINNAMON FLAX GOODNESS

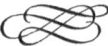

*P*rep time: 10 mins., total time: 10 min.
Serves: 3

Ingredients:
- tsp honey
- tsp cinnamon
- 2 tsp flax seed, ground
- 1 cup vanilla yogurt
- 1 tbsp. Granola
- cup flaked almonds, toasted

Instructions:
1. Thoroughly mix the honey, cinnamon, flax seed and yogurt
2. Arrange the yogurt, almonds, and granola in a jar
3. Garnish with honey and almond

Nutritional information:

Calories 88, fat 3.9g, cholesterol 5mg, sodium 59mg, carbs. 9.8g, dietary fiber 1.2g, sugars 7.4g, protein 6.2g

APPLE FLAX WRAPS

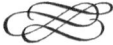

*P*rep time: 10 mins., Total time: 10 min.
Serves: 5

Ingredients:
- cup peanut butter
- 3 whole wheat tortillas
- cup apple, finely chopped
- cup shredded carrot
- cup grain-free granola
- 2 tbsp. Flaxseed, ground

Instructions:
1. Put 2 tablespoons peanut butter on each side of the tortilla
2. Drizzle the flax, granola, carrot, and apple on the tortillas
3. Fold up, split into two equal parts; serve

*N*UTRITIONAL INFORMATION:

Calories 204, fat 10.2g, cholesterol 0mg, sodium 147mg, carbs. 22.4g, dietary fiber 4.4g, sugars 5.2g, protein 7.3g

BANANA FLAX PANCAKES

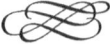

*P*rep time: 10 mins., cook time: 5 min., total time: 15 min.

Serves: 3

Ingredients:

- 2 ripe banana
- 1 large egg
- 2 servings egg whites
- 3 tbsp. Flaxseed Meal

Instructions:

1. Pour the ingredients in a blender, crack the egg into the mixture

2. Blend the mixture to smooth consistency

3. Place sprayed skillet over medium heat

4. Measure cup of the egg mixture into the hot skillet

5. Cook each side of the batter till crispy

6. Transfer to a cooling rack

7. Repeat with the remaining egg mixture

. . .

Nutritional information:

Calories 142, fat 4.2g, cholesterol 62mg, sodium 48mg, carbs. 20.3g, dietary fiber 4g, sugars 10g, protein 6.7g

ALMOND BERRY CREAM

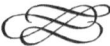

*P*rep time: 15 mins., cook time: 5 min., total time: 20 min.

Serves: 4

Ingredients:
- cup rolled oats, chopped
- cup almonds, chopped
- 3 tbsp. Flaxseeds, ground
- 1 cup plain yogurt
- 1 tbsp. Packed brown sugar
- 2 tsp vanilla extract
- 1 cup raspberries

INSTRUCTIONS:

1. Toast the chopped rolled oats and almonds over medium heat in a skillet

2. Stir constantly for 3 minutes till light brown

3. Transfer to a bowl; allow to cool. Add the Flaxseeds and stir thoroughly

4. Briskly mix the vanilla, sugar, and yogurt in a separate bowl

5. Pour this mixture into the flaxseed mixture and divide the whole mixture into four tall glasses

6. Cover each glass; refrigerate to cool. Serve cold

NUTRITIONAL INFORMATION:

Calories 209, fat 9.2g, cholesterol 4mg, sodium 46mg, carbs. 21.4g, dietary fiber 6g, sugars 8.8g, protein 8.7g

PUMPKIN MUFFINS

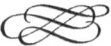

*P*rep time: 15 mins., cook time: 12 mins., total time: 27 min.

Serves: 4

Ingredients:

- 1 cup pumpkin puree
- 5 oz. Vanilla yogurt
- 1 cup gluten-free rolled oats
- 3 large eggs
- 1 tbsp. Brown sugar
- 2 tbsp. Flaxseed, ground
- 2 tsp ground cinnamon
- 1 tsp nutmeg, ground
- 2 tsp baking powder
- 1 tsp baking soda
- tsp Himalayan salt

INSTRUCTIONS:

1. Blend all ingredients till completely smooth
2. Measure cup per batter into a lightly greased muffin tin

3. Bake at 400 degrees F till edges are crispy (about 12 minutes)

4. Transfer from oven to a cooling rack (about 5 minutes)

5. Serve when cooled!

NUTRITIONAL INFORMATION:

Calories 225, fat 7.4g, cholesterol 142mg, sodium 546mg, carbs. 29.3g, dietary fiber 6g, sugars 7.2g, protein 11.6g

OAT FLAX PANCAKES WITH CREAM CHEESE

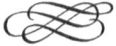

*P*rep time: 10 mins., cook time: 15 total time: 25 min.
Serves: 5

Ingredients:

- cup ground oats
- 1 cup whole wheat flour
- 3 tbsp. Flaxseed, ground
- 2 tsp baking soda
- tsp baking powder
- tsp salt
- 2 tbsp. Cocoa powder
- tsp red food coloring
- 3 egg whites
- 1 cup club soda
- 1 tbsp. Olive oil

For cream cheese topping:

- 2 tbsp. Non-fat plain Greek yogurt
- 1 tsp powder sugar
- cup unsweetened almond milk

. . .

INSTRUCTIONS:

1. Mix the main ingredients in a large bowl to your desired smooth consistency. Note: the longer the batter sits, the more fluid the oats will soak up

2. Swirl the oil in a hot pan and measure 1/4 cup of dough into it

3. Cook till you observe bubbles on the batter's surface

4. Once the bottom is crispy, flip to cook the other side (about one minute); repeat till all the dough are exhausted

Preparing the topping:

5. Combine all topping ingredients to a smooth consistency

6. Top the cream cheese mixture over the pancakes and serve

Pro tip: freeze any leftover pancakes

NUTRITIONAL INFORMATION:

Calories 216, fat 8.9g, cholesterol 0mg, sodium 666mg, carbs. 26.2g, dietary fiber 5.8g, sugars 1.3g, protein 7.9g

OAT BRAN MUFFINS

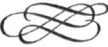

*P*rep time: 15 mins., cook time: 20 min., total time: 35 min.

Serves: 5

Ingredients:
- cup whole wheat flour
- cup coconut flour
- 1 cup ground flaxseed
- 1 oz. oat bran
- cup brown sugar, packed
- 3 tsp baking soda
- 2 tsp baking powder
- tsp salt
- 3 tsp ground cinnamon
- 1 cup carrot, thinly sliced
- cup pineapple, drained
- cup raisins
- 3 eggs
- 2 cup skim milk
- tbsp. Lemon juice
- 3 tbsp. Unsweetened applesauce

• 2 tsp vanilla

INSTRUCTIONS:

1. Combine the cinnamon, salt, baking powder, baking soda, brown sugar, oat bran, ground flaxseed and the flours in a large bowl

2. Stir in the raisins, pineapple, and carrots

3. In a separate bowl, mix the vanilla, applesauce, lemon juice, milk, and eggs

4. Stir the dry ingredients with the wet ingredients

5. Pour batter in a non-stick sprayed muffin tin

6. Bake till golden brown (about 20 minutes)

NUTRITIONAL INFORMATION:

Calories 431, fat 10.4g, cholesterol 100mg, sodium 1059mg, carbs. 69.8g, dietary fiber 9.9g, sugars 47.1g, protein 13.4g

FLAX SPICE CAKE MUFFINS

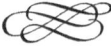

*P*rep time: 10 mins., cook time: 25 min., total time: 35 min.

Serves: 5

Ingredients:
- box spice cake mix
- cup pumpkin pie mix
- cup ground flaxseed
- cup raisins

Instructions:
1. In a large bowl, mix all ingredients completely
2. Split into greased muffin tins
3. Bake at 300 degrees F for 25 minutes

NUTRITIONAL INFORMATION:
Calories 225, fat 2.5g, cholesterol 0mg, sodium 378mg, carbs. 49.7g, dietary fiber 3.3g, sugars 22.3g, protein 3g

APPLE BANANA FLAX BALLS

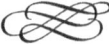

*P*rep time: 20 mins., cook time: 0 min., total time: 20 min.

Serves: 4

Ingredients:
- 2 tsp lemon juice
- cup apple, minced
- 3 tbsp. Almond butter
- cup corn flakes, crushed
- cup oats, finely ground
- cup chopped dates
- 4 tbsp. Unsweetened coconut, shredded
- 3 tbsp. Ground flaxseed

INSTRUCTIONS:

1. Mix one teaspoon lemon juice and apple in a bowl. In a separate bowl, thoroughly mix another one teaspoon lemon juice and banana

2. Puree a combination of the almond butter, banana, and dates

3. Mix the puree with the other ingredients in a mixing bowl

4. Create golf-like balls from spoonful of the mixture. Roll each ball in shredded coconut. Serve chilled!

Nutritional information:

Calories 203, fat 10.4g, cholesterol 0mg, sodium 54mg, carbs. 25.6g, dietary fiber 5.4g, sugars 13.6g, protein 4.8g

HONEY OAT BALLS

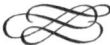

*P*rep time: 15 mins., baking time: 20 min., total time: 35 min.

Serves: 7

Ingredients:

- cup quick oats
- cup old fashioned oats
- 1 tbsp. Cocoa powder
- level scoops chocolate protein powder
- cup smooth peanut butter
- cup honey
- cup mini chocolate chips
- tsp vanilla
- 1 tbsp. Ground flaxseed
- 1 oz. Chia Seeds, Dried

INSTRUCTIONS:

1. Stir all ingredients till smooth

2. Create balls with a spoonful of the batter; place balls on a paper-lined baking sheet

3. Refrigerate for at least 15 minutes before serving

4. To serve when thawed, put balls in a zip-top bag, then, put the bag in a refrigerator

5. When it is thawed, slice and serve!

Nutritional information:

Calories 238, fat 12.1g, cholesterol 3mg, sodium 18mg, carbs. 26.3g, dietary fiber 4.5g, sugars 12.2g, protein 9g

BANANA BREAD

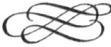

*P*rep time: 20 mins., cook time: 50 min., total time: 70 min.

Serves: 7

Ingredients:
- 2 cups coconut flour
- cup white sugar
- 3 tsp baking powder
- cup canola oil
- tsp salt
- 2 large bananas, mashed
- cup skim milk
- tsp vanilla
- cup walnuts, chopped
- 1 cup ground flax seed
- 3 small eggs

INSTRUCTIONS:

1. Mix the salt, baking powder, sugar and flour in a large bowl

2. In a separate bowl, mix the vanilla, oil, milk, eggs and mashed bananas

3. Stir in the ground flaxseed and the chopped nuts

4. Pour batter in a loaf pan coated with non-stick spray

5. Bake at 370 degrees F for 50 minutes or till dark brown

6. Transfer to a cooling rack

NUTRITIONAL INFORMATION:

Calories 412, fat 24.7g, cholesterol 59mg, sodium 157mg, carbs. 40.1g, dietary fiber 7.6g, sugars 27.6g, protein 9.2g

SOYMILK BREAD

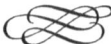

rep time: 20 mins., cook time: 45 min., total time: 65 min.

Serves: 5

Ingredients:

- cup fresh lemon juice
- cup canola oil
- cup sugar
- tsp vanilla
- 1 cup soymilk
- cup ground flaxseeds
- cup coconut flour
- 3 tsp baking powder
- tsp baking soda
- cup fresh blueberries

INSTRUCTIONS:

1. Stir the ground flaxseed, soymilk, vanilla, sugar, oil, and lemon juice in a mixing bowl

2. Add the blueberries, flour, baking powder and soda; stir thoroughly

3. Pour the mixture to a lightly oiled loaf pan

4. Bake at 375 degrees F for 45 minutes

5. Slice and serve after allowing to cool

Nutritional information:

Calories 744, fat 27g, cholesterol 0mg, sodium 225mg, carbs. 116.1g, dietary fiber 30g, sugars 67g, protein 13.2g

WHEAT FLAX BREAD

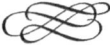

*P*rep time: 10 mins., cook time: 45 min., total time: 55 min.

Serves: 4

Ingredients:
- 2 cups water
- 2 tsp salt
- 3 tbsp. Honey
- cup ground flaxseeds
- 3 tbsp. Canola oil
- 2 cup whole wheat flour
- 3 tsp yeast

INSTRUCTIONS:

1. Use the manufacturer's instructions to measure ingredients into the bread machine pan

2. Choose "whole wheat rapid cycle."

3. Once it's completely baked (about 40 minutes), transfer to a cooling wire rack

. . .

NUTRITIONAL INFORMATION:

Calories 476, fat 17.1g, cholesterol 0mg, sodium 1175mg, carbs. 67.2g, dietary fiber 7.4g, sugars 13.4g, protein 11.1g

FLAX BUNS

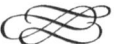

*P*rep time: 25 mins., cook time: 15 mins. Total time: 40 min.

Serves: 6

Ingredients:
- 1 tbsp. Instant yeast
- 4 cups coconut flour
- cup ground flaxseed
- cup granulated sugar
- 1 large egg
- tsp salt
- cup warm water

INSTRUCTIONS:

1. Mix the ground flaxseed, flour, and yeast in a bowl
2. In another bowl, combine the water, salt, eggs, and sugar
3. Add the flour and knead; wait for 10 minutes and punch down
4. Wait for another 10 minutes, punch down again to form buns

5. Put buns on lightly oiled baking sheet; allow 2-inch separation between the buns

6. Bake at 390 degrees F for 15 minutes; transfer to a cooling rack

7. Serve after cooling

NUTRITIONAL INFORMATION:

Calories 406, fat 11.1g, cholesterol 31mg, sodium 144mg, carbs. 64.5g, dietary fiber 34.3g, sugars 8.5g, protein 13.8g

FLAX COCONUT BREAD

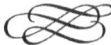

*P*rep time: 15 mins., cook time: 20 min., total time: 35 min.

Serves: 5

Ingredients:

- cup almond flour
- cup flaxseed meal
- 4 large eggs
- cup avocado oil
- tbsp. Oregano, dried and ground
- 1 tbsp. Baking powder
- 1 tsp garlic, minced
- tsp salt
- tsp rosemary
- tsp red chili flakes

INSTRUCTIONS:

1. Combine all dry ingredients in a mixing bowl

2. Stir in the wet ingredients one after the other (the olive oil should be added last)

3. Pour ingredients in an oiled baking pan
4. Bake at 390 degrees F for 20 minutes
5. Once done, cut into half squares

NUTRITIONAL INFORMATION:

Calories 197, fat 13.6g, cholesterol 149mg, sodium 415mg, carbs. 8.2g, dietary fiber 4.8g, sugars 0.5g, protein 9.7g

FLAX OATMEALS

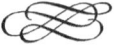

*P*rep time: 10 mins., total time: 10 min.
Serves: 4

Ingredients:

- 1 cup oatmeal
- 1 cup unsweetened almond milk
- 1 tbsp. Ground flaxseed
- 1 oz. Chia seeds
- 1 tbsp. Pure maple syrup
- tsp cinnamon
- tsp cardamon
- tsp ginger
- tsp nutmeg
- tsp vanilla

INSTRUCTIONS:

1. Puree all ingredients with a high-speed blender
2. Pour into a large container; cover then, refrigerate till morning

3. Stir in the morning; top with your favorite toppings

NUTRITIONAL INFORMATION:

Calories 240, fat 7g, cholesterol 0mg, sodium 90mg, carbs. 38g, dietary fiber 8g, sugars 6g, protein 8g

HONEY OATS ENERGY MEAL

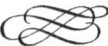

*P*rep time: 15 mins., total time: 15 min.
Serves: 7

Ingredients:
- 2 cups old fashioned oats
- cup ground flaxseed
- 1 cup cinnamon peanut butter
- cup honey
- 1 tsp vanilla extract
- 1 tsp ground cinnamon
- 1 package mini chocolate chips

INSTRUCTIONS:

1. Stir to complete smoothness all the ingredients in the order in which the ingredients are listed above

2. Create balls from the dough

3. If not ready to eat, store balls in the airtight container of your refrigerator

· · ·

NUTRITIONAL INFORMATION:

Calories 531, fat 22.9g, cholesterol 0mg, sodium 68mg, carbs. 66.3g, dietary fiber 9.9g, sugars 26.9g, protein 15.9g

QUINOA APPLE OATMEAL

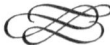

*P*rep time: 10 mins., cook time: 15 min., total time: 25 min.

Serves: 4

Ingredients:
- cup oatmeal, gluten-free
- 1 cup cooked quinoa
- 2 cups almond milk
- tsp sea salt
- 1 tsp ground cinnamon
- 1 apple, thinly sliced
- 2 tbsp. Ground flaxseed
- 2 tbsp. Walnut
- 2 tbsp. Maple syrup

INSTRUCTIONS:

1. Bring to boil a combination of the ground cinnamon, salt, milk, quinoa, and oatmeal

2. Cook over low heat to desired consistency and most liquid is completely absorbed

3. Stir in the thinly sliced apple and the Flaxseeds

4. Transfer to serving bowl; garnish with the walnut and maple syrup

NUTRITIONAL INFORMATION:

Calories 570, fat 35.4g, cholesterol 0mg, sodium 257mg, carbs. 57.1g, dietary fiber 9.5g, sugars 16g, protein 11.9g

BANANA OATMEAL

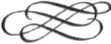

*P*rep time: 5 mins., baking time: 5 min., total time: 10 min.

Serves: 3

Ingredients:
- 1 very ripe banana, well chopped
- 1 oz. Chia seeds
- cup rolled oats
- tsp cinnamon
- cup almond milk
- cup water
- tbsp. Ground Flaxseeds

INSTRUCTIONS:

1. Combine the milk, cinnamon, oats, chia and mashed banana in a medium bowl, add water; stir again till well mixed

2. Cover and refrigerate all-night

3. Add the ground flax to the oat mixture; simmer over low heat in the morning

4. Stir constantly to desired thickness; if desired, split into portions

5. Top each portion with your favorite garnishing!

NUTRITIONAL INFORMATION:

Calories 222, fat 11.3g, cholesterol 0mg, sodium 7mg, carbs. 27.7g, dietary fiber 7.6g, sugars 5.9g, protein 5.5g

HONEY ALMOND OATS

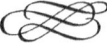

*P*rep time: 20 mins., total time: 20 min.
Serves: 7

Ingredients:

- cups oats
- cup espresso butter
- tbsp. ground almond butter
- cup honey
- 1 cup ground flaxseed
- cup chocolate chips
- 1 tsp vanilla
- 1 cup coconut flakes

INSTRUCTIONS:

1. Puree all the ingredients
2. Refrigerate for 20 minutes
3. Create 2-inch balls from the refrigerated mixture
4. Serve!

. . .

NUTRITIONAL INFORMATION:

Calories 420, fat 16g, cholesterol 8mg, sodium 23mg, carbs. 60.5g, dietary fiber 9.2g, sugars 34.2g, protein 9.1g

PEACH BLUEBERRY OATMEAL

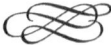

*P*rep time: 10 mins., cook time: 5 min., total time: 15 min.

Serves: 3

Ingredients:
- 1 cup oatmeal
- 2 cups water
- 2 cups fresh peaches, minced and divided
- 1 cup fresh blueberries, divided
- 1 tsp vanilla extract
- tsp cinnamon
- 1 tbsp. Ground flaxseed
- 1 tbsp. Almond butter

INSTRUCTIONS:

1. In a small saucepan, mix the cinnamon, vanilla, cup blueberries, cup peaches, water, and oatmeal

2. Cook over medium-high heat to desired consistency and thickness (about 5 minutes)

3. Pour into serving bowl; top with the nut butter, ground flaxseed, the unused peaches, and the unused blueberries

NUTRITIONAL INFORMATION:

Calories 220, fat 6g, cholesterol 0mg, sodium 8mg, carbs. 37g, dietary fiber 6.8g, sugars 14.9g, protein 6.5g

NUT SOYMILK OATMEAL

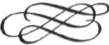

*P*rep time: 15 mins., cook time: 15 min., total time: 30 min.

Serves: 5

Ingredients:

- 2 packet gluten-free oatmeal
- 4 cups soy milk
- 2 tbsp. Maple syrup
- 1 tsp vanilla extract
- tbsp. Unrefined sugar
- 1 tbsp. Coconut oil
- 2 tsp cinnamon
- 2 medium apples, minced
- 2 tbsp. Flaxseed
- cup chopped walnuts
- 2 scoop vanilla protein powder

INSTRUCTIONS:

1. Bring to boil with medium heat, a combination of the

maple syrup, vanilla extract, soy milk, and oatmeal; stir constantly

2. Simmer for till oats are soft (about 5 minutes); set aside

3. Cook over medium heat a combination of the coconut oil, cinnamon, sugar and apples for 7 minutes; frequently stir till the apples are soft

4. In a separate bowl, mix the oatmeal, protein powder, flax, nuts, and apples

5. Combine all the mixtures to desired smoothness and thickness

6. Pour in a glass container, cover and refrigerate for at least 24 hours or at most five days

NUTRITIONAL INFORMATION:

Calories 373, fat 12g, cholesterol 1mg, sodium 204mg, carbs. 46g, dietary fiber 6.8g, sugars 27.7g, protein 21.5g

MUSO CELERIAC SOUP

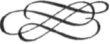

$\mathcal{P}$rep time: 15 mins., cook time: 10 min., total time: 25 min.

Serves: 2

Ingredients:
- white onion, thinly sliced
- cup celeriac, thinly sliced
- 1 tbsp. Dried Dill
- tbsp. White miso paste
- zucchini, thinly sliced
- tbsp. Lemon juice
- tsp Himalayan crystal salt
- tbsp. Avocado, minced
- 2 tbsp. Flaxseed oil
- tsp garlic powder
- stalk celery, thinly sliced
- 1 cup water

Toppings:
- tsp paprika
- 1 cup fresh herbs

. . .

INSTRUCTIONS:

1. Blend all ingredients using a high-speed blender
2. Add water and spices to desired thickness and taste
3. Pour in a soup bowl; top with the toppings
4. If desired, warm over low heat

NUTRITIONAL INFORMATION:

Calories 116, fat 3.9g, cholesterol 0mg, sodium 1223mg, carbs. 16g, dietary fiber 5.9g, sugars 5.7g, protein 6.1g

FLAX CHEESE AND CHICKEN BROTH SOUP

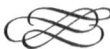

*P*rep time: 20 mins., cook time: 15 min., total time: 35 min.

Serves: 4

Ingredients:

- 1 red bell pepper, minced
- 1 tbsp. Avocado oil
- onion, thinly sliced
- 1 tsp garlic, chopped
- cup ground flaxseed
- 2 oz. Canadian bacon
- 18 oz. Chicken broth
- 3 oz. Cheddar cheese, minced

INSTRUCTIONS:

1. Bring to broil the minced red bell peppers

2. Sauté the broiled and minced red bell peppers, garlic, onion, and bacon (till onion is translucent) in a pot of oil heated over medium heat. About five minutes

3. Stir in the flax, chicken broth, and cheese

4. Pour everything in a blender and pulse

5. Pour puree in a pot and heat for 5 minutes over low heat

NUTRITIONAL INFORMATION:

Calories 165, fat 10.4g, cholesterol 29mg, sodium 740mg, carbs. 5.3g, dietary fiber 1.7g, sugars 2.3g, protein 11.9g

FLAX VEGGIE SOUP

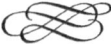

*P*rep time: 15 mins., cook time: 30 min., total time: 45 min.

Serves: 5

Ingredients:

- medium size leek, rinsed and thinly sliced
- 1 garlic clove, chopped
- 1 lb. Red potatoes, rinsed and cubed
- cup tomatoes, diced
- cup frozen green peas
- 1 bay leaf
- sprigs Parsley Raw
- tbsp. Sage
- tbsp. Rosemary, Dried
- tsp fresh thyme
- bell pepper
- large carrot, thinly sliced
- tbsp. Black peppercorns
- 1 tbsp. Paprika
- tbsp. Ground flaxseeds
- serving vegetable stock

- 1 tsp avocado oil
- tsp sea salt

INSTRUCTIONS:

1. Cook the leek (till it wilts) in a pot soup containing the avocado oil and tsp salt

2. Stir in the garlic, carrots, thyme, oregano, peppercorns, bay leaves, parsley stalks, paprika, potatoes, bell pepper, and tomatoes

3. Add water to cover mixture by a few inches; simmer

4. Add salt and cook for 10 minutes or till potatoes are tender

5. Lower the heat; stir in the flax and the green peas

6. Cover for 10 minutes to allow the peas spread into the hot broth

7. Serve or top with fresh watercress before serving!

NUTRITIONAL INFORMATION:

Calories 104, fat 0.9g, cholesterol 0mg, sodium 210mg, carbs. 22.1g, dietary fiber 4.2g, sugars 3.6g, protein 3.5g

COMPLETE VEGGIES SOUP

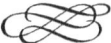

*P*rep time: 15 mins., cook time: 20 min., total time: 35 min.

Serves: 1

Ingredients:

- large onion, minced
- 1 tbsp. Avocado oil
- tbsp. Ginger, chopped
- 2 tbsp. crumbled Bay Leaf
- cup carrots, minced
- cup green beans, minced
- cup kale leaves, minced
- 2 small green onions, thinly sliced
- 1 tomato, thinly sliced
- tsp pepper powder
- 1 tbsp. Ground Flaxseeds
- 2 cup water
- tsp sea salt

INSTRUCTIONS:

1. Sauté onions in hot oil over high heat till golden brown
2. Stir in the ginger, bay leaves, minced tomato, beans, and carrots
3. Add the 2 cups of water
4. Cover and cook veggies to doneness
5. Stir in the minced kale leaves and cook for one more minute
6. Stir in the green onions and pepper powder; add salt to taste and cook one additional minute
7. Stir in the ground Flaxseeds
8. If desired, top with shredded cheese before serving

NUTRITIONAL INFORMATION:

Calories 135, fat 4.7g, cholesterol 0mg, sodium 569mg, carbs. 20.9g, dietary fiber 7.4g, sugars 6.2g, protein 4.2g

FLAX MANGO SOUP

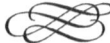

*P*rep time: 10 mins., cook time: 5 min., total time: 15 min.

Serves: 3

Ingredients:

- 1 mango, peeled and chopped
- 2 tbsp. Flaxseed, roasted and ground
- tsp chili pepper
- 1 cup water
- tbsp. Rum
- 2 ice cubes
- 1 tbsp. Cream cheese

Instructions:

1. Pulse all the ingredients using a high-speed blender
2. Pour mixture into a soup pot, add the cream cheese, and simmer over medium heat for 5 minutes
3. Serve warm!

NUTRITIONAL INFORMATION:

Calories 109, fat 3.1g, cholesterol 4mg, sodium 15mg, carbs. 18.2g, dietary fiber 3.1g, sugars 15.4g, protein 2.1g

LENTIL AND ORZO FLAX SOUP

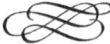

*P*rep time: 20 mins., cook time: 60 min., total time: 80 min.

Serves: 7

Ingredients:
- cup butter
- 2 small onions, thinly sliced
- 2 carrots, thinly sliced
- 2 celery stalks, minced
- 1 green pepper, minced
- 7 cups water, boiled
- cup low-sodium, chicken soup base
- 4 tsp garlic clove, chopped
- 2 tbsp. crumbled Bay Leaf
- 4 tsp Worcestershire sauce
- 38 oz. Chopped tomatoes with spices
- oz. orzo pasta
- cup lentils, dried and rinsed
- 2 tsp ground sugar
- cup ground flaxseed

. . .

INSTRUCTIONS:

1. Use medium heat to melt butter in a large pot

2. Sauté the green pepper, celery, carrot, and onion in the melted butter

3. Stir in the lentils, orzo, spiced tomatoes, Worcestershire sauce, bay leaf garlic, and the soup base

4. Add boiling water and simmer till lentils are softened

5. Stir in the sugar and flaxseed; serve!

Nutritional information:

Calories 471, fat 23.7g, cholesterol 44mg, sodium 649mg, carbs. 51.8g, dietary fiber 12.2g, sugars 11.7g, protein 11.2g

FLAX EGG COOKIES

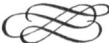

*P*rep time: 10 mins., baking time: 10 min., total time: 10 min.

Serves: 6

Ingredients:

- cup butter
- cup sugar
- 2 large eggs, separated
- 12 tsp vanilla
- 2 cups coconut flour
- 3 tbsp. Ground flaxseed
- 2 egg whites, frothy after whisking
- cup jelly

Instructions:

1. Add beaten egg yolk and vanilla to a fluffily mixed butter and sugar

2. Stir in the flour; form balls from the mixture. Dip balls in the egg white then, roll in the ground flaxseed

3. Arrange on cookie sheet; bake at 300 degrees F for 10 minutes

4. Once baked, fill in the center with the jelly

NUTRITIONAL INFORMATION:

Calories 459, fat 17g, cholesterol 89mg, sodium 117mg, carbs. 64g, dietary fiber 17.2g, sugars 30.9g, protein 9.5g

FLAX OATMEAL COOKIES

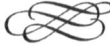

*P*rep time: 10 mins., baking time: 15 min., total time: 25 min.

Serves: 5

Ingredients:

- cup butter
- cup granulated sugar
- cups ground flaxseed
- 3 eggs
- 2 tsp vanilla
- 1 cup coconut flour
- 2 tbsp. Baking soda
- 1 cup oatmeal
- 1 tsp salt

Instructions:

1. Mix the flaxseed, butter, and sugar in a bowl
2. Stir in the beaten eggs and vanilla
3. Stir in the remaining ingredients
4. Create balls from the dough, flatten and layer on a cookie sheet

5. Bake at 400 degrees F for 10 minutes
6. Transfer to a cooling rack; serve

NUTRITIONAL INFORMATION:
Calories 418, fat 21.9g, cholesterol 131mg, sodium 2104mg, carbs. 44g, dietary fiber 14.3g, sugars 14.1g, protein 10.9g

FLAX MAPLE SYRUP OATMEAL COOKIES

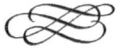

*P*rep time: 10 mins., baking time: 10 min., total time: 20 min.

Serves: 5

Ingredients:

- 1 tbsp. peanut butter
- 1 cup maple syrup
- 1 cup sugar
- 1 cup and 2 tbsp. Ground flaxseed
- cup and 5 tbsp. Soy milk
- 4 tsp vanilla
- 5 cups oatmeal, uncooked
- 2 cups whole wheat pastry flour
- 2 tsp baking soda
- 1 tsp sea salt
- 2 cups raisins

INSTRUCTIONS:

1. Mix to creamy the sugar, syrup, and peanut butter in a large bowl

2. Stir in the vanilla, soymilk and the ground flaxseed

3. Thoroughly mix the salt, baking soda, flour, and oatmeal in a separate bowl

4. Mix this mixture with the peanut butter mixture

5. Stir in the raisins; once the mixture is smooth, form meatballs

6. Put spoonful of dough on cookie sheets

7. Bake at 350 degrees F till golden brown (about 10 minutes)

8. Transfer to a cooling rack

NUTRITIONAL INFORMATION:

Calories 750, fat 8.1g, cholesterol 0mg, sodium 670mg, carbs. 159.1g, dietary fiber 11.8g, sugars 81.9g, protein 14.5g

FLAX CHUNK COOKIES

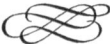

*P*rep time: 45 mins., baking time: 10 min., total time: 25 min.

Serves: 6

Ingredients:

- cup and 2 tbsp. Ground flaxseed
- cup water
- cup oats
- cup coconut flour
- 2 tsp baking soda
- tsp sea salt
- 1 cup butter
- cup natural peanut butter
- tsp brownulated sugar
- 2 tbsp. maple syrup
- 2 tsp vanilla extract
- 4 oz. Vegan baking chips

INSTRUCTIONS:

1. Briskly mix the water and one tablespoon ground flax in a small bowl; set aside, then, prepare the remaining ingredients

2. Mix the salt, baking soda, 1/3 cup ground flaxseed, oats and flour in another bowl

3. Pulse the vanilla, flax mixture, syrup, brown sugar, peanut butter, and butter

4. Mix the dry ingredients with the peanut butter mixture; stir in the chocolate

5. Split dough into two equal portions; refrigerate for 30 minutes

6. Form about 2-inch diameter balls with the dough and place on a greased baking sheet; flatten them slightly

7. Bake at 300 degree F till puffed and soft (about 10 minutes); switch off the heat, wait for 5 minutes, then, transfer to a cooling rack

NUTRITIONAL INFORMATION:

Calories 535, fat 40.7g, cholesterol 81mg, sodium 1007mg, carbs. 32.8g, dietary fiber 8.3g, sugars 6.6g, protein 11g

FLAX CAROB CHIPS COOKIES

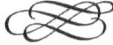

*P*rep time: 20 mins., baking time: 10 min., total time: 30 min.

Serves: 7

Ingredients:

- cup canola
- cup sugar
- cup brown sugar
- 1 large egg
- tsp vanilla
- 1 cup coconut flour
- cup oatmeal
- cup ground flaxseed
- tsp salt
- tsp baking soda
- tsp baking powder
- 1 oz. carob chips
- cup almonds, minced

Instructions:

1. Beat eggs and vanilla into creamed canola and sugars

2. Combine the baking soda, baking powder, salt, ground flaxseed, oatmeal and flour

3. Stir in the creamed mixture, almonds and carob chips in that order until it forms a smooth consistency

4. Put 1-inch balls of dough on ungreased cookie sheet with about 2-inch separation between the cookies

5. Bake at 375 degrees F for 10 minutes

NUTRITIONAL INFORMATION:

Calories 435, fat 26g, cholesterol 27mg, sodium 191mg, carbs. 45.7g, dietary fiber 10g, sugars 26.4g, protein 7.2g

FLAX WALNUT COOKIES

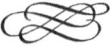

Prep time: 20 mins., baking time: 10 min., total time: 30 min.

Serves: 5

Ingredients:
- cup butter
- cup white sugar
- cup brown sugar
- cup strong cold coffee
- 1 small egg
- cup raisins
- 1 cup coconut flour
- cup walnuts, minced
- cup ground flaxseed
- tsp baking soda
- tsp sea salt
- tsp cinnamon
- tsp nutmeg

Instructions:
1. Mix all the ingredients to smooth consistency

2. Create 2-inch balls and put on an ungreased cookie sheet with 2-inch separation between them

3. Bake at 350 degrees F for 10 minutes or till you can touch without leaving an indentation

NUTRITIONAL INFORMATION:

Calories 423, fat 22.5g, cholesterol 52mg, sodium 242mg, carbs. 49.4g, dietary fiber 13.4g, sugars 26.8g, protein 9.4g

CANOLA OATMEAL COOKIES

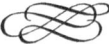

*P*rep time: 15 mins., baking time: 12 min., total time: 27 min.

Serves: 6

Ingredients:

- cup canola
- cup sugar
- cup brown sugar
- 1 large egg
- tsp vanilla
- 1 cup all-purpose unbleached flour
- cup oatmeal, powdered
- cup ground flaxseed
- tsp salt
- tsp baking powder
- 1 oz. butterscotch chips
- 1 square chocolate, thinly sliced
- cup almond, minced

Instructions:

1. Apart from the chocolate, almonds and butterscotch chips, mix the remaining ingredients to smooth consistency

2. Pulse the thinly sliced chocolate, almonds, and butter-scotch chips

3. Stir the chocolate mixture in the mixture of the other ingredients; pulse to form a smooth dough

4. Create 2-inch balls and put on an ungreased cookie sheet with 2-inch separation between them

5. Bake at 300 degrees F for 12 minutes

NUTRITIONAL INFORMATION:

Calories 550, fat 29.7g, cholesterol 31mg, sodium 134mg, carbs. 65.9g, dietary fiber 4.6g, sugars 33g, protein 9.6g

FLAX GINGERBREAD COOKIE

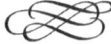

*P*rep time: 10 mins., baking time: 10 min., total time: 10 min.

Serves: 3

Ingredients:

- cup almond butter
- cup sesame seeds
- cup high protein oats
- cup unsweetened coconut, finely shredded
- tbsp. ground flaxseed meal
- tsp ground cinnamon
- tsp ginger, minced
- tsp cloves, minced
- tsp sea salt
- cup maple syrup

INSTRUCTIONS:

1. Stir all the ingredients in a mixing bowl till mixture is sticky and smooth

2. Refrigerate mixture till firm (about 10 minutes)

3. Create 1-inch balls from 1 tbsp. Of the batter using damp hands

4. Repeat till you exhaust the batter

5. Serve balls immediately or chilled

Nutritional information:

Calories 120, fat 6.9g, cholesterol 0mg, sodium 124mg, carbs. 13.7g, dietary fiber 2.6g, sugars 8.4g, protein 2.8g

FLAXSEED CHIPS

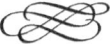

*P*rep time: 15 mins., cook time: 25 min., total time: 40 min.

Serves: 3

Ingredients:

- cup flaxseed meal, ground
- 1 tsp garlic powder
- 1 tsp onion powder
- 1 tsp chili powder mix
- 1 cup water

INSTRUCTIONS:

1. Mix the flax meal, seasonings, and water till well combined; set aside for 10 minutes

2. After 10 minutes, roll dough between two parchment papers

3. Pull away the parchment paper from the sides of the dough to prevent the paper from sticking to the dough

4. Line the rolled dough on a baking sheet and cut thickly with a pizza cutter

5. Bake for 15 minutes, remove crackers from oven, break them, spread them on a baking tray and bake for ten more additional minutes

6. Wait for cookies to cool before serving

NUTRITIONAL INFORMATION:

Calories 105, fat 5.9g, cholesterol 0mg, sodium 12mg, carbs. 6.7g, dietary fiber 5.2g, sugars 0.8g, protein 3.7g

FLAX CARROT MUFFINS

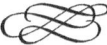

*P*rep time: 20 mins., cook time: 25 mins., total time: 45 min.

Serves: 7

Ingredients:
- 3 tbsp. Flaxseeds, ground
- 1 cup water
- 2 cups gluten-free flour blend
- cup oat flour
- 2 tsp baking powder
- 1 tsp baking soda
- tsp salt
- tsp cinnamon, ground
- tsp ground nutmeg
- tsp ginger, ground
- cup coconut oil, melted
- tsp vanilla extract
- cup plain unsweetened apple sauce
- 2 tsp freshly grated ginger
- 1 cup coconut sugar
- 2 cup carrots, chopped

• 1 tbsp. Raisins

Instructions:

1. Briskly mix the ground Flaxseeds and water; set aside to thicken

2. In a separate bowl, briskly mix the ginger, nutmeg, cinnamon, salt, baking soda, baking powder, and oat flour

3. In another bowl, stir the thick flax mixture, the freshly grated ginger, applesauce, vanilla, coconut oil, and the coconut sugar

4. Thoroughly mix the wet and dry mixture to form a smooth mixture

5. Stir in the raisins and the carrots properly

6. Split the mixture between 12 muffin cups

7. Bake at 400 degrees F for 15 minutes

NUTRITIONAL INFORMATION:

Calories 279, fat 9.4g, cholesterol 0mg, sodium 254mg, carbs. 46.2g, dietary fiber 7g, sugars 2.8g, protein 5.2g

CHOCOLATE FLAX CHIPS

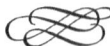

*P*rep time: 10 mins., cook time: 2 min., total time: 12 min.

Serves: 7

Ingredients:

- cup coconut, shredded, unsweetened
- cup dark chocolate chips, vegan
- 1 cup flaxseed meal, ground
- cup maple syrup
- cup peanut butter
- cup dry rolled oats

INSTRUCTIONS:

1. Mix all ingredients in a large bowl
2. Create balls from the dough
3. Microwave for 2 minutes and serve warm!

NUTRITIONAL INFORMATION:

Calories 260, fat 13.1g, cholesterol 0mg, sodium 50mg, carbs. 29.2g, dietary fiber 6g, sugars 17.2g, protein 6.5g

POMEGRANATE YOGURT FLAX
SMOOTHIE

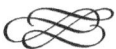

*P*rep time: 5 mins., total time: 5 min.
Serves: 3

Ingredients:
- 3 oz. Frozen blueberry
- cup pomegranate juice
- 2 tbsp. Flaxseed, ground
- 6 oz. Yogurt
- 2 bananas

INSTRUCTIONS:
Blend all ingredients till smoothly creamy

NUTRITIONAL INFORMATION:
Calories 164, fat 2.4g, cholesterol 3mg, sodium 45mg, carbs. 30.2g, dietary fiber 4.1g, sugars 19g, protein 5.2g

FLAX SCONES

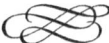

*P*rep time: 10 mins., cook time: 30 min., total time: 40 min.

Serves: 3

Ingredients:
- cup coconut flour
- cup ground flaxseed
- cup sugar
- tsp baking soda
- 3 tsp baking powder
- tsp salt
- 2 tsp cinnamon
- cup butter
- 1 cup buttermilk
- cup raisins
- 2 eggs

INSTRUCTIONS:

1. Combine the first seven ingredients to form a smooth mixture

2. Melt the butter; stir in the dry ingredients in the melted butter to form a coarse-like mixture. Stir in the buttermilk

3. Add the raisins and knead the dough till the raisins are completely incorporated

4. Roll the dough into -inch thickness

5. Create triangles of 4-inch length and 2-inch width from the dough

6. Put mixture on baking sheet, drizzle on each dough an egg white glaze

7. Bake at 390 degrees F for 20 minutes

Nutritional information:

Calories 578, fat 26g, cholesterol 153mg, sodium 579mg, carbs. 77.4g, dietary fiber 16.9g, sugars 47.2g, protein 13.4g

FLAXSEED COCONUT BARS

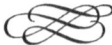

*P*rep time: 10 mins., total time: 10 min.
Serves: 5

Ingredients:
- cup maple syrup
- cup tahini
- 2 tbsp. Cocoa, ground
- 1 can dried cherries
- cup puffed rice cereal
- cup flaked coconut

INSTRUCTIONS:

1. Bring to bubble a combination of the syrup and tahini over medium heat in a large saucepan

2. Stir frequently and simmer for 2 minutes

3. Switch off the heat, stir in the cereal, cherries, flaxseed, and cocoa.

4. Use one tablespoon of mixture to create balls and roll the balls in the coconut to coat them

· · ·

Nutritional information:

    Calories 455, fat 11.1g, cholesterol 0mg, sodium 59mg, carbs. 88.3g, dietary fiber 4.3g, sugars 21.3g, protein 4.5g

FLAX BROWNIES

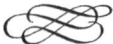

*P*rep time: 15 mins., cook time: 35 mins, total time: 45 min.

Serves: 6

Ingredients:

- cup cocoa powder
- 1 cup coconut flour
- tsp baking soda
- 1 cup sugar
- tsp salt
- cup soft tofu
- cup water
- 1 tsp pure vanilla extract
- cup ground flaxseed
- cup chocolate chips, divided, ground
- cup walnuts, thinly sliced
- 2 tbsp. Canola oil

INSTRUCTIONS:

1. Stir in the sugar and salt in a mixture of baking soda, cocoa powder, and flour

2. Pulse the tofu, water, vanilla, and ground flaxseed in a food processor

3. Add half of the ground chocolate chips to the tofu mixture and pulse to smooth consistency

4. Stir with the dry mixture, add the remaining chocolate chips

5. Mix in the canola oil till all the mixture is thoroughly mixed

6. Bake the mixture in an oiled baking pan for 35 minutes

7. Transfer to a serving plate, allow cooling before eating

NUTRITIONAL INFORMATION:

Calories 436, fat 18.3g, cholesterol 5mg, sodium 169mg, carbs. 63.6g, dietary fiber 11.8g, sugars 44.5g, protein 8g

8. APPLE CRANBERRY BAR

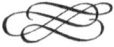

*P*rep time: 10 mins., cook time: 45 min., total time: 55 min.

Serves: 5

Ingredients:

- 3 cups baking apple, peeled and thinly sliced
- cup fresh cranberries
- 2 tbsp. Apple cider
- 1 tbsp. Brown sugar
- cup coconut flour
- 1 tbsp. All-purpose unbleached flour
- cup ground flaxseed
- cup walnuts, finely chopped
- tbsp. Wheat germ
- tsp salt
- tsp cinnamon
- 2 tbsp. Canola oil

Instructions:

1. Thoroughly mix one of tablespoon flour, sugar, cider, cranberries and apples in a bowl; pour mixture in a large baking dish

2. Combine the cinnamon, salt, wheat germ, walnuts, flaxseed, and cup flour in a separate bowl; keep stirring till the mixture is coarse

3. Evenly sprinkle the topping mixture over the fruit

4. Bake at 380 degrees F for 45 minutes or till dough is crispy

NUTRITIONAL INFORMATION:

Calories 236, fat 11.3g, cholesterol 0mg, sodium 62mg, carbs. 31.5g, dietary fiber 8.8g, sugars 17g, protein 4.3g

KRISPIES SYRUP FLAX SNACKS

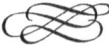

*P*rep time: 20 mins., cook time: 0 min., total time: 20 min.

Serves: 5

Ingredients:

- cup Karo corn syrup
- cup brown sugar
- cup smooth peanut butter
- cup ground flaxseeds
- tsp vanilla
- 3 cups Rice Krispies

INSTRUCTIONS:

1. Completely melt a combination of the first five ingredients over low heat in a saucepan
2. Stir in the Rice Krispies
3. Pour mixture in a large buttered sauce pan
4. Stir, flatten and cut into 5 bars.

· · ·

NUTRITIONAL INFORMATION:
Calories 360, fat 18.6g, cholesterol 0mg, sodium 91mg, carbs. 43.5g, dietary fiber 4.9g, sugars 17.6g, protein 9.6g

LEMON APPLE CRISP

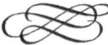

*P*rep time: 15 mins., cook time: 45 mins., total time: 60 min.

Serves: 4

Ingredients:
- 3 cups sliced apples
- tbsp. Lemon juice
- 1 tbsp. + 3 tsp white sugar
- tbsp. Cornstarch
- 1 tsp ground cinnamon
- cup ground flaxseed
- cup brown sugar, packed
- cup quick cooking oats

INSTRUCTIONS:

1. Layer a baking dish with cooking spray, toss in a combination of the apples and lemon juice till well coated
2. Blend one teaspoon cinnamon, cornstarch, and sugar
3. Stir in the apple mixture, and cornstarch mixture

4. In a separate bowl, mix the oats, brown sugar, remaining cinnamon, and ground flaxseed

5. Bake at 300 degrees F till the apples are tender and the edges are golden brown (about 45 minutes)

NUTRITIONAL INFORMATION:

Calories 179, fat 2.9g, cholesterol 0mg, sodium 6mg, carbs. 38.1g, dietary fiber 6.8g, sugars 24.6g, protein 2.5g

FLAX COCONUT CRACKERS

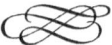

*P*rep time: 20 mins., cook time: 25 min., total time: 45 min.

Serves: 7

Ingredients:
- cup coconut flour
- cup flax seed meal
- 1 tsp salt
- cup melted coconut oil
- 1 cup coconut milk, unsweetened

INSTRUCTIONS:

1. Briskly mix the flax seed meal, salt, and coconut flour in a medium bowl

2. In a separate bowl, mix the coconut milk and coconut oil

3. Mix the wet and dry ingredients to form a smooth dough

4. Create 7-inch squares from the dough and layer on a paper-lined baking sheet; cover with another piece of parchment paper

5. Repeat till you exhaust the dough

6. Bake till all crackers are lightly browned; regularly check to remove crackers that have browned faster than the others.

7. Serve alone or with soups!

NUTRITIONAL INFORMATION:

Calories 235, fat 21.5g, cholesterol 0mg, sodium 438mg, carbs. 8g, dietary fiber 5.2g, sugars 1.3g, protein 3g

FLAX VEGGIE CRACKERS

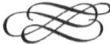

*P*rep time: 15 mins., cook time: 35 mins., total time: 50 min.

Serves: 4

Ingredients:

- cup ground flaxseed
- 1 tbsp. Chia seeds
- cup water
- tsp salt
- 3 tsp herbs and spices, dried

INSTRUCTIONS:

1. Mash water into a mixing bowl containing a mixture of all the ingredients

2. Pour spoonful of the mixture on your lined baking sheet; smoothen out each spoonful of dough

3. Cut dough to desired shapes with a sharp knife

4. Bake at 270 degrees F for 35 minutes

5. Transfer to a cooling rack; break into crackers

Pro tip: you can store in an airtight container for two weeks

NUTRITIONAL INFORMATION:
Calories 148, fat 8.8g, cholesterol 0mg, sodium 233mg, carbs. 9.8g,
dietary fiber 8.3g, sugars 0.6g, protein 5.4g

ALMOND CRACKERS

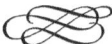

*P*rep time: 15 mins., baking time: 20 min., total time: 35 min.

Serves: 3

Ingredients:
- 2 large eggs
- tsp salt
- 1 tsp freshly ground black pepper
- cup finely ground almond flour
- cup ground flaxseed

INSTRUCTIONS:

1. Briskly mix all the ingredients to form a well-integrated dough

2. Put spoonful of dough on a piece of parchment paper, cover with another piece of parchment paper

3. Smoothen to about -inch thickness; transfer to a baking pan sprayed with baking powder

4. Bake at 300-degree F till crackers turn golden brown (about 20 minutes)

5. When it is baked, transfer to a cooling rack

6. Once cooled, transfer an airtight bag for storage.

Pro tip: the crackers around the edges will brown quicker than those at other places, so, ensure you regularly check to prevent burnt crackers.

NUTRITIONAL INFORMATION:

Calories 190, fat 13.2g, cholesterol 124mg, sodium 443mg, carbs. 6.9g, dietary fiber 4.9g, sugars 0.4g, protein 9.3g

FLAX OATS BALLS

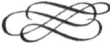

*P*rep time: 40 mins., total time: 40 min.
Serves: 5

Ingredients:

- cup natural peanut butter
- cup dry oats
- cup ground flaxseed
- cup chocolate chips
- cup honey
- tsp ground cinnamon

INSTRUCTIONS:

1. Thoroughly combine all the ingredients in a medium bowl
2. Cover and refrigerate until firm (about 30 minutes)
3. Form 1-inch diameter balls with a scoop of the dough
4. Store balls in the fridge for 3 days using an airtight container

. . .

NUTRITIONAL INFORMATION:

Calories 247, fat 13.3g, cholesterol 2mg, sodium 12mg, carbs. 24.7g, dietary fiber 3.8g, sugars 14.8g, protein 8.1g

FLAX HONEY ENERGY BITES

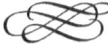

*P*rep time: 25 mins., total time: 25 min.
Serves: 4

Ingredients:

- 1 tbsp. creamy natural peanut butter
- cup honey
- 1 tsp cinnamon
- tsp salt
- 3 cups oats
- oz. Chia Seeds, Dried
- cup unsweetened coconut, minced
- cup flaxseed meal
- cup chocolate chips

Instructions:

1. Briskly mix the cinnamon, honey and peanut butter in a medium bowl; stir in the salt

2. Stir in the flaxseed, coconut, chia seeds and oats to smooth consistency

3. Stir in the chocolate chips

4. Create 2-inch balls with a scoop of the batter

5. Serve at once or chilled!

NUTRITIONAL INFORMATION:

Calories 654, fat 23.1g, cholesterol 5mg, sodium 319mg, carbs. 97.9g, dietary fiber 13.7g, sugars 48.8g, protein 15.1g

STRAWBERRY OAT PROTEIN BALLS

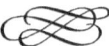

*P*rep time: 15 mins., total time: 15 min.
Serves: 5

Ingredients:

- cup peanut butter
- cup raw honey
- tsp vanilla
- cup vanilla protein powder
- cup ground flaxseed meal
- cup unsweetened coconut, minced
- cup rolled oats
- oz. Chia Seeds, Dried
- cup dried strawberries, thinly sliced

INSTRUCTIONS:

1. Thoroughly combine all the ingredients in the order listed
2. Create balls with a spoonful of the mixture
3. Store in an airtight container; serve immediately or freeze for 1 week

. . .

Nutritional information:

Calories 180, fat 9.6g, cholesterol 2mg, sodium 74mg, carbs. 16.2g, dietary fiber 3.6g, sugars 9g, protein 9.8g

CONCLUSION

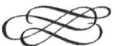

*R*emember these words of Franklin D. Roosevelt: *"Men are not prisoners of fate, but prisoners of their minds."*

You know what? He was right. So, are you a prisoner of your mind? Or have you broken free of its constraints?

Congratulations! You now know all you need to know about using flaxseeds to prevent breast cancer and solve gut problems. Indeed, if universities handed out PhDs in this field, you'd have one by now! Yes, just knowing all these secrets is quite an accomplishment.

But the truth is, packing away all this information in your noggin won't do you any good if you don't put it to use. And that's why I suggest you take action – starting right now – by preparing the smoothies and start consuming them. Even if you start with any of the recipes, you're sure to get great results either way - why not try it for yourself and see?